Understanding Achalasia

The Perfect Self Care Guide To Achalasia Cure, Treatment, Management And Recovery For Your Complete Wellness

Dr. Travis Nicholas

Contents

CHAPTER ONE 3
   Achalasia 3
   Who Receives Achalasia? 5
   Is Achalasia Serious? 6
   What Motives Achalasia? 12

CHAPTER TWO 15
   What Are The Signs And Symptoms Of Achalasia? 15
   Management And Treatment 20
   Balloon Dilation 24
   Medication 25
   Esophagectomy 27
   Treatments For Achalasia Include 32

CHAPTER THREE 35
   What Is The Definition Of Achalasia? 35
   How Is Esophageal Feature Unusual In Achalasia? 39
   What Motives Achalasia? 44
   What Assessments Do Medical Doctors Use To Diagnose Achalasia? 47
   What Is The Remedy For Achalasia? 61

Diagnosis 62

CHAPTER FOUR 67

Treatment 67

Risk Factors 78

Outlook 80

Swallowing Disorders 93

THE END 95

CHAPTER ONE

Achalasia

What is achalasia?

Achalasia is a uncommon however serious circumstance that impacts your esophagus, the tube that incorporates meals from your throat to your stomach.

With achalasia, your decrease esophageal sphincter (LES) fails to open up at some point of swallowing. This muscular ring closes off your esophagus from your belly most of the time, however it opens when you swallow so meals can ignore through. When it doesn't open, meals can again up inside your esophagus.

Symptoms of this circumstance have a tendency to come on gradually, and they can get worse as time goes on. Eventually, it can come to be challenging to swallow beverages or food, however therapy can help.

Who Receives Achalasia?

Achalasia is a pretty uncommon condition. According to 2021 lookup

In the United States, about 1 in each and every 100,000 humans increase the circumstance every year

Elsewhere in the world, between 0.1 to 1 in each and every 100,000 human beings advance the circumstance every year

This circumstance seems to have an effect on human

beings of all genders at roughly the identical rates. It's much less frequent in children: of achalasia instances are identified in youth beneath the age of 16.

While adults of any age can get achalasia, it most many times develops after age 30 and earlier than age 60.

Is Achalasia Serious?

Without treatment, achalasia can purpose serious fitness complications, including:

Megaesophagus. This refers to an enlarged and weakened esophagus.

Esophagitis. This refers to inflammation and infection in your esophagus.

Esophageal perforation. A gap can structure in the partitions of your esophagus if they emerge as too susceptible from backed-up food. If this happens, you'll want scientific cure proper away to stop infection.

Aspiration pneumonia. This takes place when the particles of meals and liquid trapped in your esophagus enter your lungs

Achalasia can additionally enlarge your possibilities of creating esophageal cancer.

There's no remedy for achalasia, so even with treatment, your signs may also no longer go away entirely. You may additionally want to have a couple of tactics and make everlasting way of life changes, including:

Eating smaller meals

Avoiding any ingredients that reason heartburn

Quitting smoking, if you smoke

Sleeping propped up as an alternative of mendacity flat

Without treatment, achalasia can motive serious fitness complications, including:

Megaesophagus. This refers to an enlarged and weakened esophagus.

Esophagitis. This refers to infection and infection in your esophagus.

Esophageal perforation. A gap can shape in the partitions of your esophagus if they end up too susceptible from backed-up food. If this happens, you'll want clinical remedy proper away to forestall infection.

Aspiration pneumonia. This takes place when the particles

of meals and liquid trapped in your esophagus enter your lungs

Achalasia can additionally expand your probabilities of creating esophageal cancer.

There's no remedy for achalasia, so even with treatment, your signs and symptoms can also no longer go away entirely. You may also want to have a couple of tactics and make everlasting life-style changes, including:

Eating smaller meals

Avoiding any ingredients that motive heartburn

Quitting smoking, if you smoke

Sleeping propped up as a substitute of mendacity flat

What Motives Achalasia?

Why your esophageal muscular tissues fail to contract and relax generally is unknown. One principle is that achalasia is an autoimmune disorder (your physique assaults itself) that is prompted by means of a virus. Your immune machine assaults the nerve cells in the muscle layers of the partitions of your esophagus and at the LES. Your nerve cells, which manage muscle function, slowly degenerate for motives that are now not presently understood. This effects in immoderate contractions in the LES. If you have achalasia, the LES fails to loosen up and meals and beverages can't pass by via your esophagus into your stomach.

A uncommon shape of achalasia might also be inherited. More lookup is needed.

CHAPTER TWO

What Are The Signs And Symptoms Of Achalasia?

Achalasia signs and symptoms increase slowly, with signs and symptoms lasting for months or years. Symptoms include:

Trouble swallowing (dysphagia). This is the most frequent early symptom.

Regurgitation of undigested food.

Chest ache that comes and goes; ache can be severe.

Heartburn.

Cough at night

Weight loss/malnutrition from problem eating. This is a late symptom.

Hiccups, issue belching (less frequent symptoms)

What are the issues of achalasia?

Some problems of achalasia are the end result of meals backing up (regurgitating) into your esophagus and then drawn into (aspirated) your trachea (windpipe), which leads to your lungs. These problems include:

Pneumonia.

Lung infections (pulmonary infections).

Other issues include:

Esophageal cancer. Having achalasia will increase your hazard of this cancer.

How is achalasia diagnosed?

Three checks are usually used to diagnose achalasia:

Barium swallow: For this test, you'll swallow a barium guidance (liquid or different form) and its motion thru your esophagus is evaluated the use of X-rays. The barium swallow will exhibit a narrowing of the esophagus at the LES.

Upper endoscopy: In this test, a flexible, slim tube with a digital camera on it – known as an endoscope – is handed down your esophagus. The digicam tasks pix of the interior of your esophagus onto a display for evaluation. This check helps rule out cancerous (malignant) lesions as nicely as check for achalasia.

Manometry: This take a look at measures the timing and power of your esophageal muscle contractions and rest of the decrease esophageal sphincter (LES). Failure of the LES to loosen up in response to swallowing and lack of muscle contractions alongside the partitions of the esophagus is a high-quality check for achalasia. This is the "gold standard" take a look at for diagnosing achalasia.

Management And Treatment

How is achalasia treated?

Several redress are accessible for achalasia such as nonsurgical choices (balloon dilation, medications, and botulinum toxin injection) and surgical options. The aim of therapy is to relieve your signs with the aid of enjoyable your decrease esophageal sphincter (LES).

Your healthcare company will talk about these preferences so you each can determine the nice remedy for you primarily based on the severity of your situation and your preferences.

Minimally Invasive Surgery

The surgical procedure used to deal with achalasia is known as laparoscopic esophagomyotomy or laparoscopic Heller myotomy. In this minimally invasive surgery, a thin, telescopic-like instrument known as an endoscope is inserted thru a small incision. The endoscope is related to a tiny video digital camera – smaller than a dime –that tasks a view of the operative website onto video video display units positioned in the working room. In this operation, the muscle fibers of the LES are cut. The addition of some other technique referred to as a partial fundoplication helps forestall gastroesophageal reflux, a aspect impact of the Heller myotomy procedure.

Peroral endoscopic myotomy (POEM) is a minimally invasive choice to laparascopic Heller myotomy. In this procedure, muscle tissue on the aspect of the esophagus, the LES and the top phase of the belly are reduce with a knife. The cuts in these areas loosen the muscles, permitting the esophagus to empty like it generally should, passing meals down into your stomach.

Balloon Dilation

In this non-surgical procedure, you'll be put underneath mild sedation whilst a particularly designed balloon is inserted thru the LES and then inflated. The manner relaxes the muscle sphincter, which lets in meals to enter your stomach. Balloon dilation is normally the first remedy choice in human beings in whom surgical procedure fails.

You can also have to bear a number of dilation remedies to relieve your symptoms, and each and every few years to preserve relief.

Medication

If you aren't a candidate for balloon dilation or surgical treatment or pick now not to endure these procedures, you may additionally gain from Botox® (botulinum toxin) injections. Botox is a protein made via the micro organism that motive botulism. When injected into muscle mass in very small quantities, Botox can loosen up spastic muscles. It works by way of blocking off the sign from the nerves to the sphincter muscle tissues that inform them to contract. Injections want to be repeated to preserve symptom control.

Other remedy redress encompass nifedipine (Procardia XL®, Adalat CC®) or isosorbide (Imdur®,

Monoket®). These medicines loosen up the spastic esophageal muscle tissues by way of reducing LES pressure. These remedies are much less wonderful than surgical treatment or balloon dilation and furnish only momentary comfort of your symptoms.

Esophagectomy

Removal of your esophagus is a remaining lodge treatment.

What are the problems of redress for achalasia?

Complications of achalasia redress include:

Creation of a gap in the esophagus.

Lack of success and return of achalasia symptoms.

Gastroesophageal reflux disease.

Bloating.

What post-treatment follow-up is needed?

Long-term follow-up is wished regardless of which

cure you receive. This is due to the fact redress are palliative – which means they relieve signs – and do no longer treatment achalasia or halt its progression. Symptoms can return. Your healthcare issuer will favor to see if your esophagus is thoroughly permitting meals to enter your belly and to test for gastroesophageal reflux, which would want to be treated. Your physician will additionally choose to reveal you to be certain most cancers has no longer developed.

Facts you have to comprehend about achalasia

Achalasia is a uncommon disorder of the muscle of the decrease esophageal physique and the decrease esophageal sphincter that prevents leisure of the sphincter and reduces contractions, or peristalsis, of the esophagus.

The reason of achalasia is unknown; however, there is degeneration of the esophageal muscle mass and, greater importantly, the nerves that manipulate the muscles.

Common signs of achalasia include

Difficulty in swallowing (dysphagia),

Chest pain, and

Regurgitation of meals and liquids.

Complications of achalasia consist of lung troubles and weight loss.

Achalasia can also enlarge the threat of most cancers of the esophagus, however this no longer nicely established.

Achalasia can be recognized through X-ray, endoscopy, or esophageal manometry.

Treatments For Achalasia Include

Oral medications,

Dilation or stretching of the esophagus,

Surgery (open and laparoscopic),

Endoscopic surgery, and

Injection of muscle-relaxing drug treatments (botulinum toxin) at once into the esophagus.

There is no unique weight loss program to deal with achalasia. However, some sufferers analyze what ingredients appear to bypass thru the esophagus extra easily, and make dietary variations to consist of these ingredients in their diet, for example:

Drinking liquid foods

Drinking greater water with meals, and

Drinking carbonated drinks (the carbonation looks to assist "push" the meals via the esophageal sphincter).

If a individual with achalasia has weight loss that is substantial; their weight-reduction plan may also be supplemented via a liquid food plan that is whole (contains all crucial vitamins to stop malnutrition).

CHAPTER THREE

What Is The Definition Of Achalasia?

Achalasia can be described as the lack of the decrease esophageal sphincter to loosen up and the presence of atypical motility in the the rest of the esophagus.

How does the regular esophagus function?

The esophagus has three practical parts. The uppermost section is the higher esophageal sphincter, a specialised ring of muscle that varieties the top give up of the tubular esophagus and separates the esophagus from the throat. The top sphincter stays closed most of the time to forestall meals in the major section of the esophagus from backing up into the throat. The fundamental phase of the esophagus is referred to as the physique of the esophagus, a long, muscular tube about 20 cm (8 in) in length. The 0.33 purposeful section of the esophagus is the decrease esophageal sphincter, a ring of specialised esophageal muscle at the junction of the esophagus with the stomach. Like the higher sphincter, the decrease sphincter stays closed most of the time to stop meals and acid from backing up into the physique of the esophagus from the stomach.

The higher sphincter relaxes with swallowing to permit meals and saliva to omit from the throat into the esophageal body. The muscle in the higher esophagus simply under the top sphincter then contracts, squeezing meals and saliva in addition down into the esophageal body. The ring-like contraction of the muscle progresses down the physique of the esophagus, propelling the meals and saliva toward the stomach. (The development of the muscular contraction via the esophageal physique is referred to as a peristaltic wave.). By the time the peristaltic wave reaches the decrease sphincter, the sphincter has opened, and the meals passes into the stomach.

How Is Esophageal Feature Unusual In Achalasia?

In achalasia, there is an incapability of the decrease sphincter to loosen up and open to let meals bypass into the stomach. In at least 1/2 of the patients, the lower sphincter resting stress (the strain in the decrease sphincter when the affected person is now not swallowing) additionally is abnormally high. In addition to the abnormalities of the decrease sphincter, the muscle of the decrease half of to two-thirds of the physique of the esophagus does no longer contract normally, that is, peristaltic waves are much less usual or forceful and, therefore, meals and saliva are no longer propelled down the esophagus and into the stomach. A few sufferers with achalasia have very high-pressure contractions in the decrease esophageal physique following swallows, however these high-pressure waves are no longer superb in pushing meals into the stomach. These sufferers are referred to as having "vigorous" achalasia. These abnormalities of the decrease sphincter and esophageal physique are accountable for meals sticking in the esophagus.

Achalasia is considered as consisting of three levels or

types. The earliest stage or kind is regarded to be when the sphincter does no longer open appropriately, and the contractions of the decrease esophageal physique are susceptible or intermittent. Dysphagia is regularly mild, and sufferers research how to modify their consuming habits to get round the problem. If caught at this stage and dealt with appropriately, it is believed that the prognosis is first-rate and later ranges may additionally be prevented. Over time besides treatment, it is believed that the destruction of the nerves and muscle mass as properly as the obstruction posed by means of the sphincter leads to the improvement of failure of the esophageal muscle to generate contractions and esophageal dilation, regarded a 2d kind of achalasia. Vigorous achalasia is regarded a 1/3 type. In addition to sphincter dysfunction, excessive stress contractions or spasms occur, which are per chance an strive to overcome the obstruction induced through the tight sphincter. The esophagus frequently is no longer significantly dilated.

What Motives Achalasia?

The purpose of achalasia is unknown. Theories on causation invoke infection, heredity or an abnormality of the immune gadget that reasons the physique itself to injury the esophagus (autoimmune disease).

The esophagus incorporates each muscular tissues and nerves. The nerves coordinate the rest and opening of the sphincters as nicely as the peristaltic waves in the physique of the esophagus. Achalasia has outcomes on both the muscular tissues and nerves of the esophagus; however, the outcomes on the nerves are believed to be the most important. Early in achalasia, infection can be considered (when a scientific expert examines esophageal tissue below the microscope) in the muscle of the decrease esophagus, particularly round the nerves. As the sickness progresses, the nerves start to degenerate and in the end disappear, specially the nerves that reason the decrease esophageal sphincter to relax. Still later in the development of the disease, muscle cells start to degenerate, perchance due to the fact of the injury to the nerves. The result of these modifications is a decrease sphincter that can't loosen up and muscle in the decrease esophageal physique that can't guide peristaltic waves. With time, the physique of the esophagus stretches and turns into enlarged (dilated).

What Assessments Do Medical Doctors Use To Diagnose Achalasia?

The analysis of achalasia frequently is suspected on the groundwork of the history. Patients typically describe a innovative (worsening) of swallowing (dysphagia) for strong and liquid meals over a duration of many months to years. They may also word regurgitation of food, chest pain, or loss of weight. Rarely, the first symptom is aspiration pneumonia.

Because sufferers commonly research to compensate for their dysphagia by using taking smaller bites, chewing well, and consuming slowly, the analysis of achalasia regularly is delayed via months or even years. The lengthen in prognosis of achalasia is unlucky due to the fact it is believed that early cure -- earlier than marked dilation of the esophagus takes place -- can forestall esophageal dilation and its complications.

The dysphagia in achalasia additionally is special from the dysphagia of esophageal stricture (narrowing of the esophagus due to scarring) and esophageal cancer. In achalasia, dysphagia typically takes place with each stable and liquid food, whereas in esophageal stricture and cancer, the dysphagia usually happens solely with stable food and now not liquids, till very late in the development of the stricture. The innovative worsening of the dysphagia, specially with cancer, is greater rapid.

X-ray studies

The analysis of achalasia generally is made with the aid of an X-ray learn about known as a video-esophagram in which video X-rays of the esophagus are taken after barium is swallowed. The barium fills the esophagus, and the emptying of the barium into the belly can be observed. In achalasia, the video-esophagram indicates that the esophagus is dilated (enlarged or widened), with a attribute tapered narrowing of the decrease end, every so often likened to a "bird's beak." In addition, the barium stays in the esophagus longer than regular earlier than passing into the stomach.

Esophageal manometry

Another test, esophageal manometry, can display particularly the abnormalities of muscle characteristic that are attribute of achalasia, that is, the failure of the muscle of the esophageal physique to contract with swallowing and the failure of the decrease esophageal sphincter to relax. For manometry, a skinny tube that measures the strain generated via the contracting esophageal muscle is exceeded via the nose, down the returned of the throat and into the esophagus. In a affected person with achalasia, no peristaltic waves are considered in the decrease 1/2 of the esophagus after swallows, and the strain inside the gotten smaller lower esophageal sphincter does now not fall with the swallow. In sufferers with lively achalasia, a robust simultaneous contraction of the muscle may additionally be viewed in the decrease esophageal body. An gain of manometry is that it can diagnose achalasia early in its path at a time at which the video-esophagram may also be normal.

Endoscopy

Endoscopy additionally is useful in the prognosis of achalasia though it can be ordinary early in achalasia. Endoscopy is a system in which a bendy fiberoptic tube with a mild and digital camera on the cease is swallowed. The digicam presents direct visualization of the inner of the esophagus. One of the earliest endoscopic findings in achalasia is resistance as the endoscope is handed from the esophagus and into the belly due to the excessive strain in the decrease esophageal sphincter. Later, endoscopy might also expose a dilated esophagus and a lack of peristaltic waves. Endoscopy additionally is necessary due to the fact it excludes the presence of esophageal most cancers and different reasons of dysphagia.

Two stipulations can mimic achalasia, esophageal most cancers and Chagas' sickness (Chagas) of the esophagus. Both can provide upward jostle to video-esophageal and manometric abnormalities that are indistinguishable from achalasia. Fortunately, endoscopy normally can leave out the presence of cancer. If there is greater concern, computerized tomography (CT) or magnetic resonance imaging (MRI) of the lowermost esophagus can be executed to perceive cancers close to the decrease esophageal sphincter.

Chagas' disorder is an contamination induced by way of the parasite, Trypanosoma cruzi, and is restricted to Central and South America. It is surpassed to people via insect bites from the reduviid bug. The parasite is shed in the bug's feces at the time it is biting. Scratching the chunk breaks the pores and skin and permits the parasite to enter the body. The parasite spreads all through the physique however takes up predominant residency in the muscle tissues of the gastrointestinal tract, from the esophagus to the rectum, even though it additionally frequently influences the muscle of the heart. In the gastrointestinal tract, the parasite motives degeneration of the nerves controlling the muscle groups and can lead to unusual feature somewhere in the gastrointestinal tract. When it impacts the esophagus, the abnormalities are equal to these of achalasia.

Acute Chagas' ailment happens in general in children. In these men and women who are considered at a a lot later time for issues of swallowing, the acute sickness is long-gone. The prognosis of Chagas' sickness can be suspected if there is involvement of different components of the gastrointestinal tract, such as dilation of the small gut or the colon, and the heart. The fantastic approach for making a prognosis is through serological checks searching for antibodies in the blood in opposition to the parasite.

What Is The Remedy For Achalasia?

Treatments for achalasia consist of oral medications, stretching of the lower esophageal sphincter (dilation), surgical procedure to reduce the sphincter (esophagomyotomy), and the injection of botulinum toxin (Botox) into the sphincter. All 4 remedies decrease the stress inside the decrease esophageal sphincter to enable simpler passage of meals from the esophagus into the stomach.

Diagnosis

Achalasia's rarity can complicate analysis of the condition, due to the fact some docs may additionally no longer straight away apprehend the signs.

A health practitioner or different healthcare expert (HCP) would possibly suspect you have achalasia if you:

Have hassle swallowing each solids and beverages and this situation worsens over time

Experience regurgitation of food

Have heartburn, chest pain, or both

They may also use a few exclusive strategies to assist diagnose the condition:

Endoscopy. In this procedure, a gastroenterologist will insert a tube with a small digicam on the cease into your esophagus to seem for symptoms of achalasia. This take a look at solely leads to analysis in about a thirdtrusted Source of achalasia cases, however an endoscopy can assist rule out different conditions, like belly or esophageal cancer.

X-ray. An X-ray of your chest can exhibit whether or not your esophagus is enlarged and preserving meals trapped inside. A health practitioner or different HCP may additionally additionally endorse a barium swallow for the x-ray. Taking liquid barium earlier than your X-ray makes it feasible for them to music how the liquid strikes down your esophagus.

Esophageal manometry (motility study). For this test, a gastroenterologist will pass by a slim tube into your esophagus via your nose. The tube will measure stress as you swallow, revealing how the muscle tissues of your esophagus work and whether or not any stress has constructed up at the LES.

The order of these diagnostic assessments can also rely on your unique signs and household history, however docs frequently advise an endoscopy first.

Some evidencetrusted Source suggests esophageal manometry is the most dependable diagnostic tool, as this check can diagnose achalasia extra than ninety percentage of the time.

CHAPTER FOUR

Treatment

Achalasia therapy can't totally remedy the condition, however it can help:

Improve your capability to swallow by way of opening the LES

Reduce different symptoms, like ache and regurgitation

Lower the possibilities of an abnormally enlarged esophagus

Possible redress include:

Pneumatic dilation

This nonsurgical cure includes passing a exclusive balloon into the decrease section of your esophagus and then inflating it. The balloon helps stretch out the muscular tissues of your LES, increasing the opening so meals can omit via greater easily.

This method isn't besides risk, though. Dilation can now and again lead to esophageal perforation, a pretty amazing however serious complication.

A perforation can be repaired, however if this happens, you'll want surgical treatment proper away.

For about 30 percenttrusted Source of people, signs will in the end return, so you would possibly want this remedy once more in the future.

You're extra in all likelihood to want repeat remedies if you:

Were assigned male at birth

Are youthful than forty years old

Have respiratory concerns

Have already had the system at least once

Botox injections

Another nonsurgical option, this process includes injections of botulinum toxin (Botox) into your esophagus at some point of an endoscopy. A medical doctor or different HCP may also propose this cure if different redress don't assist or you pick to keep away from surgery.

Botox blocks the nerves that commonly sign your muscle groups to contract, so it can assist loosen up the LES so it opens and permits meals to omit through. These injections can enhance signs and symptoms quickly. The outcomes aren't permanent, though, so you'll want to have the remedy repeated inside about 6 months to a year.

Potential downsides encompass the price of repeated treatments, plus the truth that repeated Botox injections ought to have an effect on the later success of surgerytrusted Source.

Laparoscopic Heller myotomy

In a myotomy, a healthcare professional will reduce the LES muscle fibers to assist loosen up it so meals can bypass into your belly extra easily.

Surgeons can use laparoscopic or robotic methods to operate this surgical procedure much less invasively, thru 5 small incisions to your abdomen. You'll normally want anesthesia and an in a single day continue to be in the hospital.

This surgical procedure has a excessive success rate, however signs and symptoms of GERD can strengthen as a viable complication. The healthcare professional will probable additionally operate a system to assist stop reflux, such as a partial fundoplication.

Peroral endoscopic myotomy

This more recent technique is very comparable to a Heller myotomy, however the use of an endoscope makes it much less invasive.

The endoscopic method does have a drawback, though: It prevents the medical professional from doing a partial fundoplication at the equal time.

In different words, you have a excessive chance of experiencing GERD signs after the system and may additionally want some other remedy for GERD later on.

Medication

If you can't get surgical procedure proper away, or decide on to keep away from it if at all possible, sure medicinal drugs can provide some alleviation from your symptoms.

Medication alternatives include:

Nitrates, which assist promote rest of the easy muscle making up the decrease phase of your esophagus

Calcium channel blockers, which can assist decrease LES stress with the aid of maintaining calcium from getting into cells and disrupting muscle contractions

Sildenafil, a phosphodiesterase-5 inhibitor that can assist decrease stress in the LES, enjoyable it ample so meals can bypass through

These medicines can also contain some facet effects, including:

Low blood pressure

Head pain

Dizziness and fainting

Swelling in your legs and feet

Medications usually won't absolutely enhance your symptoms, either, so a health practitioner or different HCP will commonly solely propose them as a temporary treatment.

Risk Factors

Because of achalasia's rarity, professionals don't completely recognize how or why it occurs, or who may have a higher danger of growing the condition.

A few workable hazard elements include:

Having a spinal wire injury

Getting endoscopic sclerotherapy to deal with bleeding or enlarged veins

Having a viral infection

Having an autoimmune disease

Age — it's greater frequent in center age and older adulthood

Future lookup on achalasia may additionally assist specialists research extra about feasible elements contributing to its development, alongside with techniques that may assist forestall the condition.

Outlook

The outlook for this situation varies. Getting a prognosis faster instead than later can assist you get cure to enhance your signs earlier than they end up severe.

You may additionally want a couple of remedies earlier than your signs and symptoms improve. Keep in mind, though, that if one remedy doesn't work, you do have different choices to consider. A health practitioner or different HCP might, for example, propose surgical operation if a dilation system doesn't work.

Older lookup suggests that whilst achalasia can reason fitness complications, it doesn't show up to have a tremendous have an impact on on lifestyles expectancy.

Diet, oral medications, and botulinum toxin (Botox) to deal with achalasia

What about achalasia and diet?

There is no unique weight loss program for treating achalasia, even though dietary modifications regularly are made by way of sufferers as they research what ingredients appear to bypass greater easily. Usually, the greater liquid meals omit greater easily, and sufferers once in a while drink greater water with their meals. Early in the development of the sickness they may also locate that carbonated drinks assist meals pass, likely due to the fact of the accelerated intra-esophageal stress induced with the aid of the carbonation that "pushes" meals via the sphincter. If loss of weight is massive it is realistic to complement meals with a liquid food regimen complement that is complete, i.e., consists of all quintessential nutrients, to stop malnutrition.

Oral medications

Oral medicinal drugs that assist to loosen up the decrease esophageal sphincter encompass companies of pills referred to as nitrates, for example, isosorbide dinitrate (Isordil) and calcium channel blockers (ccbs), for example, nifedipine (Procardia) and verapamil (Calan). Although some sufferers with achalasia, in particular early in the disease, have enchancment of signs with medications, most do not. By themselves, oral medicinal drugs are probable to grant solely non permanent and now not long-term remedy of the signs of achalasia, and many sufferers trip side-effects from the medications.

Botulinum toxin

Another therapy for achalasia is the endoscopic injection of botulinum toxin into the decrease sphincter to weaken it. Injection is quick, nonsurgical, and requires no hospitalization. Treatment with botulinum toxin is safe, however the consequences on the sphincter regularly remaining solely for months, and extra injections with botulinum toxin might also be necessary. Injection is a desirable alternative for sufferers who are very aged or are at excessive danger for surgery, for example, sufferers with extreme coronary heart or lung disease. It additionally permits sufferers who have misplaced extensive weight to devour and enhance their dietary repute prior to "permanent" cure with surgery. This may additionally minimize post-surgical complications.

What consequence can I count on from the a variety of cure options?

Balloon dilation improves signs and symptoms in 50% to 93% of human beings with achalasia. Keep in thinking that the manner might also want to be repeated to hold symptom improvement. Repeated dilations make bigger the chance of inflicting a gap (perforation) in your esophagus.

Minimally invasive surgery/laparoscopic Heller myotomy is fine in 76% to one hundred percent of humans with achalasia. Keep in thinking that up to 15% of human beings journey gastroesophageal reflux signs and symptoms after surgery.

Botox injection correctly relaxes spastic esophageal sphincter muscular tissues in up to 35% of humans with achalasia. The injections ought to be repeated each and every six to 12 months to preserve symptom relief.

Medications, such as nifedipine, enhance signs in

0% to 75% of humans with achalasia; isosorbide improves signs and symptoms in 53% to 87%.

Affected Populations

Achalasia is a uncommon ailment that usually impacts adults between the a while of 25 and 60 years. However, this sickness may additionally take place at any age, such as for the duration of childhood. Achalasia impacts men and ladies in equal numbers besides in instances that show up to replicate an inherited form. In these cases, it seems that adult males are twice as probably as ladies to be recognized with this disorder.

Related Disorders

Symptoms of the following problems can be comparable to these of achalasia. Comparisons may additionally be beneficial for a differential diagnosis:

Esophageal cancer

The signs and symptoms of esophageal most cancers resemble these related with achalasia. Esophageal most cancers may additionally start at nearly any factor in the tube. Small cancers can also be asymptomatic or might also be current besides symptoms. As the tumor grows, the first signal can also be concern in swallowing and/or ache upon swallowing and/or feeling as if meals had been caught in the back of the breastbone. Difficulty in swallowing might also be accompanied by means of indigestion, heartburn and choking. Weight loss is now not uncommon.

Swallowing Disorders

Swallowing problems come in a range of forms. Some are the end result of disturbances of the talent such as Parkinson's disease, more than one sclerosis or amyotrophic lateral sclerosis (ALS or Lou Gehrig's disease). Others are the end result of malfunctioning of components of the throat worried in swallowing. For example, the pharynx may additionally malfunction after a stroke.

THE END

Made in the USA
Las Vegas, NV
05 February 2024